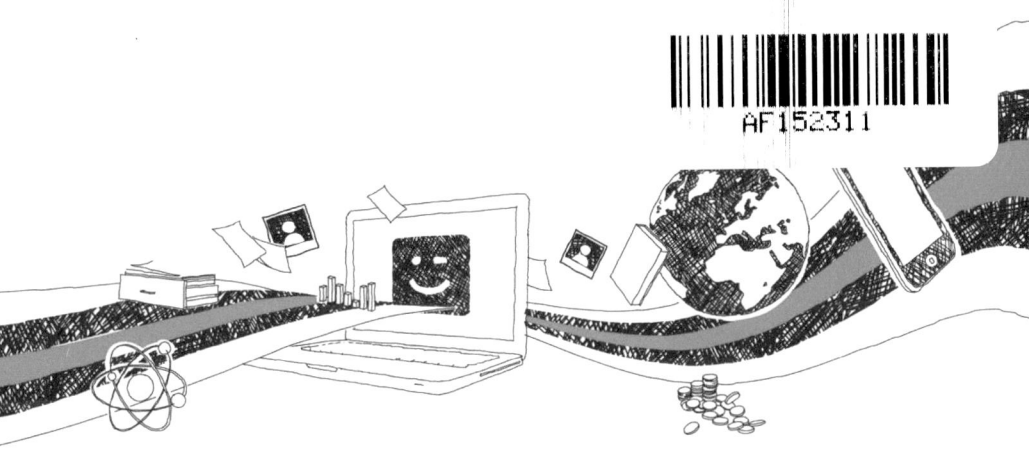
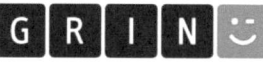

Breastfeeding in West Africa, Nigeria. A Look on its Health Benefits

Bibliographic information published by the German National Library:

The German National Library lists this publication in the National Bibliography; detailed bibliographic data are available on the Internet at http://dnb.dnb.de.

ISBN: 9783346429339
This book is also available as an ebook.

© GRIN Publishing GmbH
Nymphenburger Straße 86
80636 München

Print and binding: Books on Demand GmbH, Norderstedt, Germany
Printed on acid-free paper from responsible sources.

The present work has been carefully prepared. Nevertheless, authors and publishers do not incur liability for the correctness of information, notes, links and advice as well as any printing errors.

GRIN web shop: https://www.grin.com/document/1027075

Contents

Introduction... 2

Social Determinants of Exclusive Breastfeeding.. 3

    Economic Stability. 4

    Education.. 5

    Social and Community Context 5

    Culture and family support.. 6

    Health and Health Care 7

Implications... 8

References... 12

Introduction

Breastfeeding infants is a public health priority because of its considerable benefit and recent studies have shown that it protects the health of the infant, decreases the chances of metabolic disorders, and the rate of child mortality (IP *et al.*, 2009; Balogun, *et al.*, 2017). It is beneficial to a nursing mother, as it reduces the time for uterine involution and postpartum bleeding, reduces chances of breast and ovarian cancers and helps the mother and child to bond (Gartner *et al.*, 2005; Jernstrom, 2004). Thus, the concern of the World Health Organization (WHO) to encourage the practice in postpartum mothers and to promote Exclusive Breastfeeding (EBF) in infants from 0 to 6 months. Regarding breastfeeding, the United Nations Children's Fund (UNICEF) and the World Health Organization (WHO), suggests that newborns are exclusively breastfed throughout the earliest 6 months of their lives and the breastfeeding continued until the 24th month of age (WHO/UNICEF, 2005). However, despite the efforts to make infant formula bioequivalence of breast milk, breast milk remains the surest source of natural nutrition for infants (Imdad *et al.*, 2011). Breast milk contains bioactive factors, digestive enzymes and nutrients useful for infants' growth, development and immune defence. Several initiatives such as the Baby-Friendly Hospital was launched to promote exclusive breastfeeding. Yet, a survey by Bhattacharjee *et al.*, (2019), reported that in 2017, only 37% of newborns less than 6 months, were exclusively breastfed. This study identified an existent geospatial difference in the practice of absolute breastfeeding and reported a marked heterogeneity across countries in Africa, and the rural, suburban and urban settlements. While the report had it that 1/3 children below the age of 6 months are exclusively breastfed in developing countries, recent findings observed the practice of EBF increased from 33% to 39% from 1995 to 2010 respectively, and major progress noted in West and Central Africa (Haron *et al.*, 2013). Another investigation carried out from 2010 to

2

2015, on the prevalence of breastfeeding and it's exclusivity up until 6months of infants' age, observed that West Africa and Central Africa ranked low (Issaka *et al.*, 2017). In Nigeria, it is assumed that almost every child is breastfed, but from 1999 to 2013 there was a record of decrease (from 28% to 17%) in the prevalence of exclusive breastfeeding and a low (38%) rate of breastfeeding initiated within the first hours of the childbirth (Adewuyi and Adefemi, 2016). While several factors such as the demand of work and maternal illnesses were faulted as reasons in the decline of exclusivity in breastfeeding (Adewuyi and Adefemi, 2016), Ogbo *et al,* (2008) sampled the data of 10,225 children below the age of 2 years and recorded that, while 38% of them were predominately breastfed, 14% were exclusively breastfed. Also, the study revealed a geographical variation in breastfeeding patterns within the Country, with the Northern regions having lower prevalence compared to the other regions. A comparative study on the attitude and practice of breastfeeding done in South-western, Nigeria, had shown 57.3% of mothers in rural settlements had a more positive attitude towards breastfeeding, 75.8% had initiated breastfeeding within the first hours of delivery and 79.8% of them practised EBF compared to the 25.9% of their urban equivalents (Balogun *et al,* 2017 pp. 123-130).

Social Determinants of Exclusive Breastfeeding

Certain factors have fundamental influence over the health status of an individual, they include the political, socio-economic and cultural conditions that could mould the health status of an individual and a nation (Raphael 2008, p.2, WHO, 2008). Citing international directives on exclusive breastfeeding and its conventional advantages, this exercise is less than average in most developing countries inclusive of Nigeria (Haroon et al, 2013; Salami, 2006). In a bid to understand why EBF is at an unsatisfactory level In Nigeria, studies have been done to identify likely trends and factors (Ogbo *et al*, 2008; Ogunlesi, 2010 pp. 459-465; Agho *et al*, 2011,

Salami, 2006) and amongst identified elements, Ogbo et al, 2008, mentioned geopolitical location, finance, health services and individual factors (age of the mother, occupation and babies' gender and family condition) as some of the determinants of EBF in nursing mothers. In this review, the Healthy People 2020 approach to Social Determinants of Health (Healthy People, 2020), would be assessed in regards to the exclusive breastfeeding practices in Nigeria and these include;

- Economic Stability
- Education
- Social and Community Context
- Health and Health Care
- Neighbourhood and built Environment

Economic Stability.

Economic stability to a great extent informs the socio-economic status of an individual and the same is said of nursing mothers (Ogbo *et al*, 2015). According to previous studies, the higher the socio-economic status of the nursing mother (Agho *et al.,* 2011), the higher the tendencies of adopting EBF and as observed by Ogbo *et al.*, 2015, women from wealthier families give exclusive breastfeeding to their infants compared to their counterparts. Nonetheless, the economic stability of these nursing mothers is assessed based on employment, characterized by the presence or absence of a Job. A study by Splendor *et al*, 2019, sampled a number of first time nursing mothers, in South-Eastern Nigeria and of the 83.6% who were employed, 62.1% were to return to work 3 to 4 months after delivery. This finding supports other claims that women in public or private engagement do not breastfeed for long nor practice exclusively in breastfeeding because of the time demanded by work and the need to work due to the country's economic challenges (Agunbiade and Opeyemi, 2012; Adewuyi and Adefemi, 2016).

Education

This refers to the level of formal education attained by the nursing mother and its influence on the practice of EBF; Ogbo *et al.,* 2015, in his study, identified that among other factors in Nigeria, women with atleast a primary level of education were more likely to exclusively breastfeed their newborns than women with no formal education. Similarly, Okafor *et al*, 2012 observed that in Lagos, Nigeria, women with secondary education were 8 times more prone to exclusively breastfeed their newborns when compared with those without any formal education. Even so, Agho *et al.* (2011), correlated economic stability and level of formal education and realized that 26.1% of women with secondary education, from wealthy household practised EBF unlike the 13.7% obtained from women in poor homes and without a formal education. One of the reason suggestive of this observation is that educated mothers are inclined to follow antenatal instructions (Splendor *et al*, 2019).

Social and Community Context

Under this umbrella, the following would be discussed to understand how they influence the practice of exclusive breastfeeding in Nigeria.

Age

Some studies believed that the older the age of the mother, the more experienced she would be at breastfeeding, and the more the tendencies for her to exclusively breastfeed her newborn up until 6 months of age (Lawoyin *et al*, 2001). Similar to the findings by Ukegbu *et al*, 2011 and Qureshi *et al*, 2011, Ogbo et al, 2015 reported that mothers within the ages of 25- 34 years in South-East Nigeria are more likely to practice EBF than those below this age range.

Culture and family support

When Adegoke and Anthony (2008) studied the influence of culture on health practices in south-west Nigeria, they concluded that substantial therapeutic interventions can be effective if it acknowledges the place of culture in health practices. Fortunately, the practise of breastfeeding is embedded in the various cultures across the ethnic groups in Nigeria (Gartner *et al*, 2005), but the concern is how well EBF is embraced (Agunbiade and Oyeyemi, 2012). In a typical Nigerian culture, a child is groomed by both the mother, paternal and maternal grandmothers respectively; a practice that has significance on decisions on how and if the child is weaned. Sometimes, these other women encourage nursing mothers to give herbal concoctions to the newborns to preserve their health; a practice which relegates the place of exclusive breastfeeding and exposes the infant to contaminations (Agunbiade and Opeyemi, 2012). In North-Western Nigeria, mothers consider colostrum as dirt and harmful, and they give animal milk, water, honey, almond and wash outside from the Quran to the newborn while they wait for fresh breast milk (Oche *et al.*, 2011). Unfortunately, in South-Eastern Nigeria, Uchendu *et al* (2009), observed that about 52% of nursing women who never practised EBF, did so because of opposition from family members.

Health and Health Care

Various health care conditions, such as pregnancy care, mode of delivery and postnatal care are identified to be of influence to breastfeeding practices (Benova *et al*, n.d). While birth by traditional attendants is still a common practice in Nigeria, Agho *et al*. 2011, observed that EBF rate was higher in mothers who were delivered by professional health attendants than the traditional ones, and noted a lower rate (6.0%) of EBF exercises among nursing mothers with no prenatal care compared with the rate (23.5%) of EBF in infants born of mothers with more than 3 prenatal visits. Considering delivery by professional health workers, it is believed that on delivery at health facilities and during prenatal clinical visits, mothers have better access to information and campaigns on breastfeeding (Ukegbu *et al*, 2011; Okafor *et al*, 2014). Similar to the findings by Gawayan *et al*, 2014; Ogbo *et al*, 2015 noted that even among women with good access to health facilities and professionals, socioeconomic position and family pressures plays a bigger role in the decision of exclusive breastfeeding. It was noted that misconceptions and misinformation from these health professionals negatively affect the EBF practice. According to the study by Utoo et al, in 2012, 22.2% of health professionals in South-South Nigeria, indicated sagging of the breast as a con of breastfeeding; misinformation which could be relayed to nursing mothers and consequently discourage the practice. According to Ogbo *et al.*, 2015 and Benova *et al.* 2020, women who delivered their baby through a cesarean section are less likely to do exclusive breastfeeding.

Neighbourhood and Built Environment

As reported by several studies, there are variations in the practice rate of EBF across the geopolitical regions of Nigeria. Agho *et al*, 2011 in his study reported that EBF was least practised in the North West and North East of Nigeria. Similarly, nursing mothers from Southern Nigeria were more educated, wealthier and had better access to health facilities and more likely to be employed, thus they are more prone to early initiation of breastfeeding, yet less likely to continue exclusively due to factors such as the need to resume work by these mothers (Ogbo *et al*, 2015). In regards to the place of residence, Splendor *et al*, 2019 started that it is significantly associated with knowledge of exclusive breastfeeding and the level of knowledge EBF is significant in determining its practice (Agho *et al*, 2011). A comparison between the urban and rural community within the same geopolitical zone in South East, Nigeria revealed that 91% of urban residing nursing mothers, had the right knowledge and attitude towards exclusive breastfeeding than the 89% of rural nursing mothers (Maduforo and Onurah, 2011).

Implications

In 2018, Nigeria's Demographic and Health Survey (NDHS), revealed that across the country, only 29% of children below 6 months of age were breastfed and the average duration of excluded breastfeeding was at 2.8 months (Benova *et al*, 2020). The Baby-Friendly Hospital Initiative (BFHI), was birthed from the 1990 Innocenti Declaration and was launched in 1991, this initiative was inaugurated to encourage exclusive breastfeeding for infants from the earliest 6 months of age and sustained till 1 year of age (WHO/UNICEF, 2009). This initiative was adopted in Nigeria in 1992 (ogunlesi *et al*, 2004), and a lot of this depended on the visitation of Baby-Friendly Hospitals by the nursing mothers; Ndiokwelu *et al*, 2016 reported that 74% of mothers among the study sample were aware of exclusive breastfeeding due to information obtained from the hospital through the nurses. Despite the high level of awareness, Ndiokwelu *et al* 2016, reported that merely 31.5% of the respondents practised exclusive breastfeeding, this shows a poor result of the BFHI. Ojofetimi *et al,* 2000 discovered that BHFI existed in the Urban and rural areas of Southern, whilst more impact and response was recorded in the urban settlements than the rural, in the rural areas, most pregnant mothers are delivered of their babies at home and by traditional birth attendants (Ogbo *et al,* 2015 p. 259).

As part of the local efforts to improve infant health through nutrition, Nigeria has adopted a series of policies to enhance the EBF rates, with the inability of the BFHI to evoke a much anticipated response, the National Breastfeeding Policy was created in 1998, a policy which was put in place to give flexibility to women in the workforce (Madurofo and Onuaha, 2011), however, Wurogyi and Etuk, (2016 pp. 534-554), cited the lack of adequate legal backing to back the freedom of women to exclusively breastfed their newborns for 6 months, as employees in the labour force; and only very few states embraced the 6 months leave initiative for breastfeeding mothers (Federal Ministry of Health, 2020). With the failed attempt to improve the practice of EBF (Ogbo *et al,* 2016), in 2001, the National Policy on Food and Nutrition was adopted and then in 2005, National Policy on Infants and Young Child Feeding (Ogbo *et al,* 2016).

Yet, as of 2018, the child mortality rate was ranked at 69 deaths out of 1000 children, whereas the mortality rate of less than 5-year-old children was at 132 deaths per 1000 children (Guardian, 2019). Agho *et al,* 2011 studied the rate of EBF across various states in Nigeria and observed that Nigeria had a low practice of EBF compared to various neighbouring countries. It is worthy of note that, the cultural practices such feeding the newborns with herbs or water at the onset of birth exposed these infants to contaminations from infections and elides them of the antibiotics from colostrum thus increasing the rate of mortality and comorbidities in these infants (Agunbiade *et al,* 2012, Agho *et al*, 2011).

The International Code of Marketing of Breast milk Substitutes (the Code) adopted in 1981 by the World Health Assembly (WHA), states that breast milk substitutes should not be advertised or promoted to the public and promo samples should not be made available to the public. This codebase has seen a consistent violation in   Nigeria (Ogbo *et al*, 2016) and as part of the government effort to remedy this, it became subsidiary legislation of the National Agency for Food and Drug Administration and Control (NAFDAC) in June 2019. Since this time, the agency has languished over the growing market of these feeding substitutes and the lack of cooperation from health professionals who recommend infant formulas to mothers (Nigeria Health Watch, 2019).

The federal government of Nigeria, have launched various health campaigns to promote breastfeeding practices and one of such was the 'zero water campaign' awareness on the need for nursing mothers to desist giving water to their newborns less than 6 months of age, in celebration of 2019 world breastfeeding week. However, during the 2020 World breastfeeding week celebration involving the government and another stakeholder, the Nigerian government pledged to review the Baby-Friendly Initiative in line with WHO 10 steps guidelines, reinforced the need importance for breastfeeding during the COVID-19 pandemic and the goal to achieve 50% exclusive breastfeeding in the country by 2025 (Federal Ministry of Health, 2020).

Conclusion

Nursing mothers are faced with a lot of factors including their ability to embrace EBF wholeheartedly. Thus the need for the government to provide grassroots solutions to these problems because achieving optimal EBF in Nigeria is a necessity if the country would win the fight against child mortality and morbidity; a way to promote the sustainable development goal. There is a need for the Nigerian government and other stakeholders to incorporate the World Health Organization and UNICEF recommendation of the Baby-Friendly Community Initiative (BFCI), to increase community involvement in the practice of EBF. This practice has seen success in other countries such as Kenya and New Zealand (Ekanem and Fajola, 2016 pp. 229-230).

A noteworthy recommendation is that EBF promotion campaigns, policies and programme should be specifically targeted at mothers, from deprived backgrounds, that is, the impoverished and uneducated nursing mothers, also, traditional birth attendants should be sensitized and educated on the importance of EBF so that, women in the rural areas who utilize their services can be adequately informed.

The National Breastfeeding policy that was aimed at giving liberty to working mothers to exclusively breastfeed their infants should be strengthened and support systems such as the provision of daycare in the office space, breastfeeding breaks for mothers, paid maternal and paternal leave, longer maternal leave should be provided. Also, the implementation of the International Code of Marketing of Breast-milk Substitutes should be treated as urgent (Ogbo *et al*, 2015).

References

Adewuyi EO, Adefemi K., 2016. Breastfeeding in Nigeria: a systematic review. *Int J Community Med Public Health*, 3:385-96. Available at: https://dx.doi.org/10.18203/2394-6040.ijcmph201604217 (Accessed: 4th November, 2020)

Agunbiade, O.M., Ogunleye, O.V., 2012. Constraints to exclusive breastfeeding practice among breastfeeding mothers in Southwest Nigeria: implications for scaling up. *Int Breastfeed J* 7, 5. Available at: https://doi.org/10.1186/1746-4358-7-5 (Accessed: 6th November, 2020)

Agho, K.E., Dibley, M.J., Odiase, J.I. et al. (2011). Determinants of exclusive breastfeeding in Nigeria. *BMC Pregnancy Childbirth* 11, 2. Available at: https://doi.org/10.1186/1471-2393-11-2 (Accessed: 7th November, 2020).

Balogun M.R., Okpalugo O.A., Ogunyemi A.O., Sekoni AO. (2017). Knowledge, attitude, and practice of breastfeeding: A comparative study of mothers in urban and rural communities of Lagos, Southwest Nigeria. *Niger Med J*, 58:123-30. Available at: https://www.nigeriamedj.com/text.asp?2017/58/4/123/256997. (Accessed: 4th November, 2020)

Benova L, Siddiqi M, Abejirinde I.O 2020. Time trends and determinants of breastfeeding practices among adolescents and young women in Nigeria, 2003–2018BMJ Global Health 2020; 5: e002516. Available at:https://gh.bmj.com/content/5/8/e002516.citation-tools (Accessed: 8th November, 2020).

Bhattacharjee, N.V., Schaeffer, L.E., Marczak, L.B. et al., 2019. Mapping exclusive breastfeeding in Africa between 2000 and 2017. *Nat Med* 25, 1205–1212. Available at: https://doi.org/10.1038/s41591-019-0525-0 (Accessed: 4th November, 2020).

Chika I. Ndiokwelu, Odinakachukwu I.C. Nwosu, Peace Nwanneka Ani, Annastecia Ogechi Chizike and Maduforo Aloysius Nwabugo, 2016. Impact of the Baby Friendly Hospital Initiative (BFHI) Programme on Breast-Feeding Knowledge, Attitude and Practices of Mothers. *Pakistan Journal of Nutrition*, 15: 244-248. Available at: https://scialert.net/abstract/amp.php?doi=pjn.2016.244.248 (Accessed: 7th November, 2020).

Exclusive breastfeeding and public policies. (2019). *The Guardian* Available at:https://m.guardian.ng/opinion/exclusive-breastfeeding-and-public-policies/ (Accessed: 8th November, 2020).

Gartner LM, Morton J, Lawrence RA, Naylor AJ, O'Hare D, Schanler RJ, Eidelman A.I., 2005.Breastfeeding and the use of human milk. *Pediatrics*. 115 (2): 496-506.10.1542/peds.2004-2491.

Gayawan, E., Adebayo, S.B. & Chitekwe, S., 2014. Exclusive Breastfeeding Practice in Nigeria: A Bayesian Stepwise Regression Analysis. *Matern Child Health J* 18, 2148–2157. Available at: https://doi.org/10.1007/s10995-014-1463-6 (Accessed: 6th November 2020).

Haroon, S., Das, J.K., Salam, R.A. et al., 2013. Breastfeeding promotion interventions and breastfeeding practices: a systematic review. *BMC Public Health* 13, S20 (2013). Available at: https://doi.org/10.1186/1471-2458-13-S3-S20 (Accesses: 4th November, 2020)

Imdad, A., Yakoob, M.Y. and Bhutta, Z.A., 2011. Effect of breastfeeding promotion interventions on breastfeeding rates, with special focus on developing countries. *BMC Public Health* 11, S24. Available at: https://doi.org/10.1186/1471-2458-11-S3-S24 (Accessed: 4th November, 2020).

Ip Stanley, Chung M., Raman G., Trikalinos A.T., Lau J., 2009. A Summary of the Agency for Healthcare Research and Quality's Evidence Report on Breastfeeding in Developed Countries. Available at:https://doi.org/10.1089/bfm.2009.0050 (Accessed: 4th November, 2020).

Issaka A.I., Agho K.E., and Renzaho A.M., 2017.Prevalence of key breastfeeding indicators in 29 sub-Saharan African countries: a meta-analysis of demographic and health surveys (2010–2015). Available at: https://dx.doi.org/10.1136%2Fbmjopen-2016-014145 (Accessed: 4th November, 2020)

Jernström, H., Lubinski, J., Lynch, H. T., Ghadirian, P., Neuhausen, S., Isaacs, C., Weber, B. L., Horsman, D., Rosen, B., Foulkes, W. D., Friedman, E., Gershoni-Baruch, R., Ainsworth, P., Daly, M., Garber, J., Olsson, H., Sun, P., & Narod, S. A. (2004). Breast-feeding and the risk of breast cancer in BRCA1 and BRCA2 mutation carriers. *Journal of the National Cancer Institute*, 96(14), 1094–1098. https://doi.org/10.1093/jnci/djh211 (Accessed 4 November, 2020)

Lawoyin T.O, Olawuyi J.F., and Onadeko M.O. (2001). Factors associated with exclusive breastfeeding in Ibadan, Nigeria. *Sage Journals*. Available at: https://doi.org/10.1177/089033440101700406 (Accessed: 8th November, 2020).

Oche, M. O., & Umar, A. S. (2008). Breastfeeding practices of mothers in a rural community of Sokoto, Nigeria. *The Nigerian postgraduate medical journal*, 15(2), 101–104.Available at: (Accessed: 8th November, 2020).

Ogbo, F.A., Agho, K.E., and Page, A. 2015. Determinants of suboptimal breastfeeding practices in Nigeria: evidence from the 2008 demographic and health survey. *BMC Public Health* 15, 259. Available at: https://doi.org/10.1186/s12889-015-1595-7 (Accessed: 4th November, 2020)

Ogbo, F.A., Page, A., Idoko, J., Claudio F., Agho K., 2016. Have policy responses in Nigeria resulted in improvements in infant and young child feeding practices in Nigeria? Int Breastfeed Journal, (2)9, Available at: https://doi.org/10.1186/s13006-017-0101-5 (Accessed: 8th November 2020).

Splendor C.N., Okafor .B.C, Anarado N.A., Onuigbo N.N., Chinweuba A.U., Nwaneri A.C., Arinze J. C., Chikeme C.P., 2019. "Exclusive Breastfeeding Knowledge, Intention to Practice and Predictors among Primiparous Women in Enugu South-East, Nigeria", *Journal of Pregnancy*. Available at: https://doi.org/10.1155/2019/9832075 (Accessed: 7th November, 2020).

Utoo B., Ochejele S., Obulu M., and Utoo, P. (2012). Breastfeeding Knowledge and Attitudes amongst Health Workers in a Health Care Facility in South-South Nigeria: the Need for Middle Level Health

Manpower Development. *Clinics in Mother and Child Health*. 9. 1-5. 10.4303/cmch/235565. (Accessed: 7th November 2020).

WHO. Infant and Young Child feeding. Model Chapter for textbooks for medical students and allied health professionals. Geneva: World Health Organization, 2009.

Worugji I.N.E, and Etuk S.J. (2005). The National Breastfeeding Policy in Nigeria: The Working Mother and the Law, Health Care for Women International, 26:7, 534-554. Available at: https://10.1080/07399330591004863 (Accessed: 8th November, 2020).

YOUR KNOWLEDGE HAS VALUE

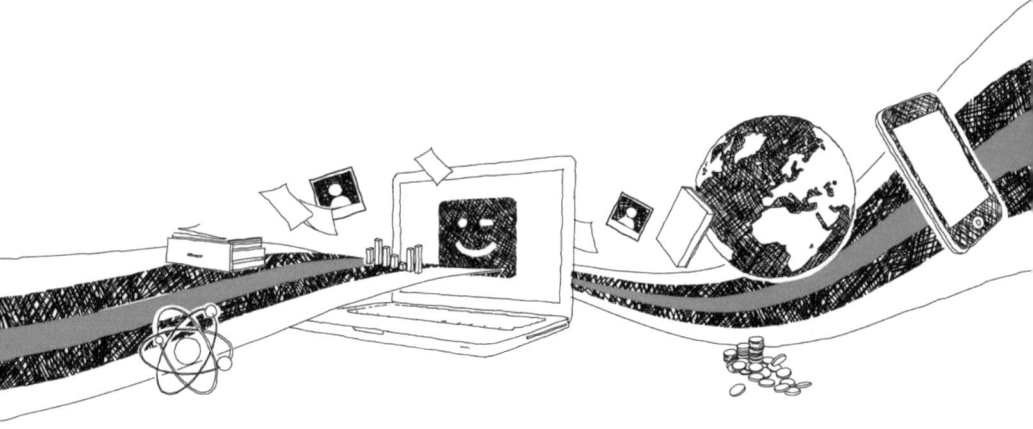

- We will publish your bachelor's and master's thesis, essays and papers

- Your own eBook and book - sold worldwide in all relevant shops

- Earn money with each sale

Upload your text at www.GRIN.com
and publish for free

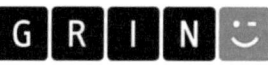